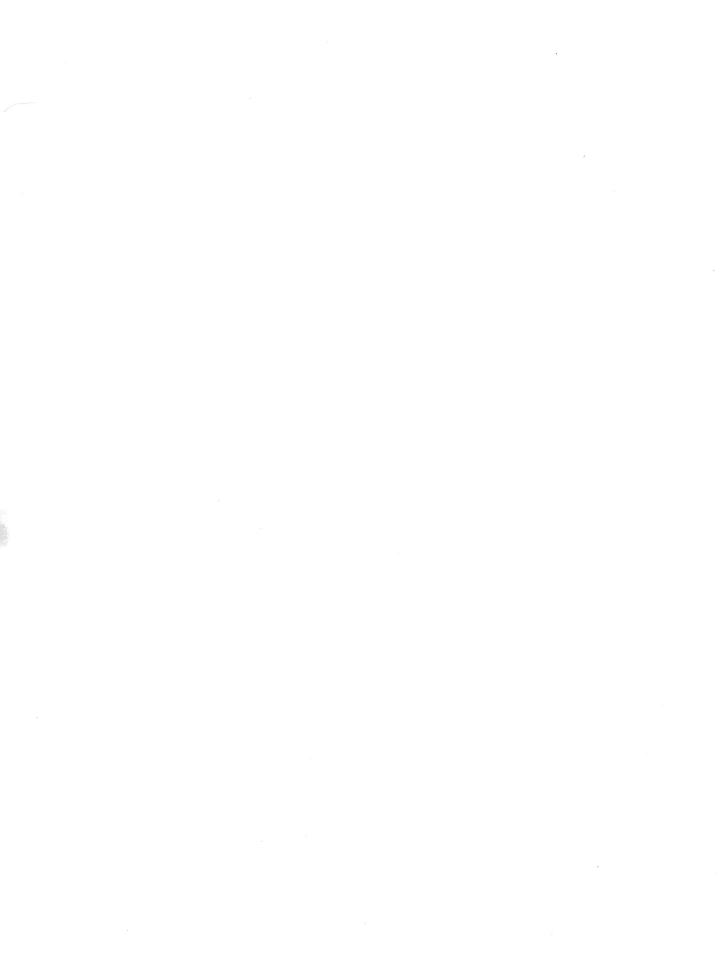

I AM LEAH STRONG

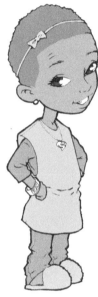

Written by Leah and Devon Still

Illustrated by Leonard Green

Published by Tiffany M. Shepard, J.D.

Written by Leah and Devon Still
Illustrated by Leonard Green
Published by Tiffany M. Shepard, J.D.

Editorial staff
Senior Editor, Marissa Wright
Shannon Cofer, BSN, RN
Karima Douglas
Erin Mason, M.ED
Holly Mech
Jaimie Miller

For more information go to IAmLeahStrong.com

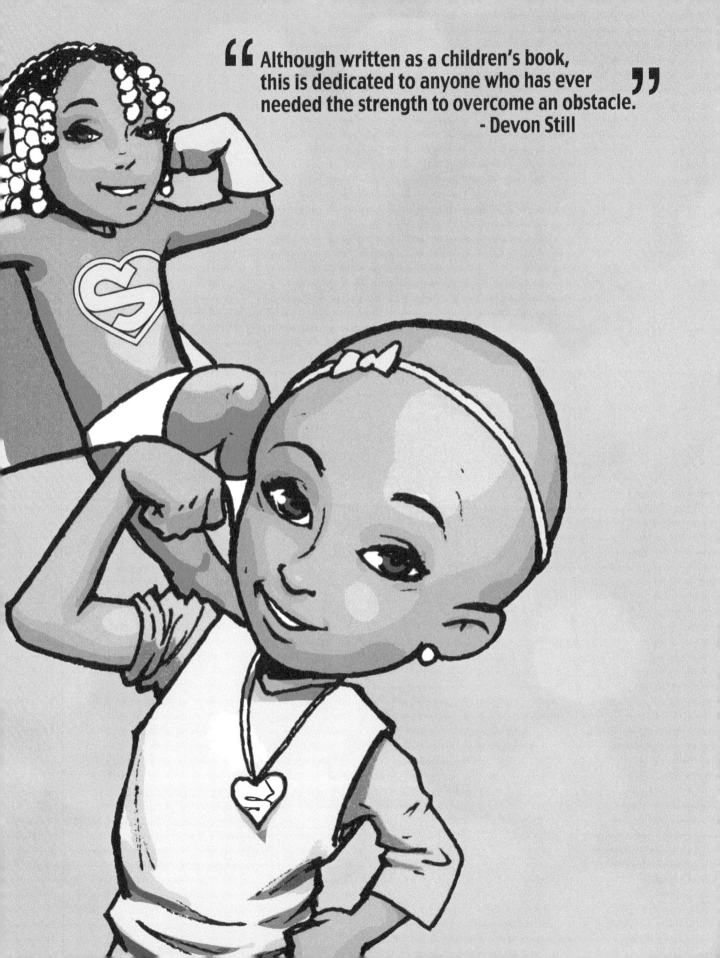

"Although written as a children's book, this is dedicated to anyone who has ever needed the strength to overcome an obstacle."
- Devon Still

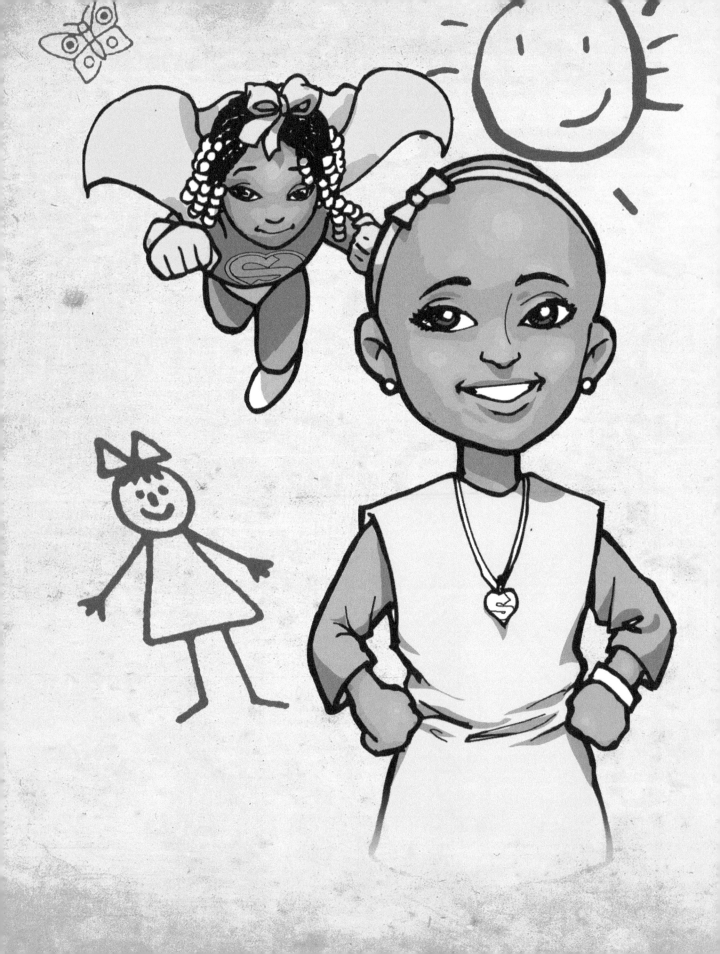

hi, my name is leah still.

when i was four years old, i was diagnosed with neuroblastoma (my dad said that's how you spell it). neuroblastoma is a type of cancer that kids can get. sitting in the hospital can sometimes be boring, so i decided to write a book to keep me busy in between my treatments. i'm here to let you know that battling cancer or any other disease can be a very scary process but with the support of my friends and family, i stayed strong... i was still strong... i am leah strong. and i'm here to tell you, you are strong too!

love, leah still

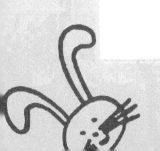

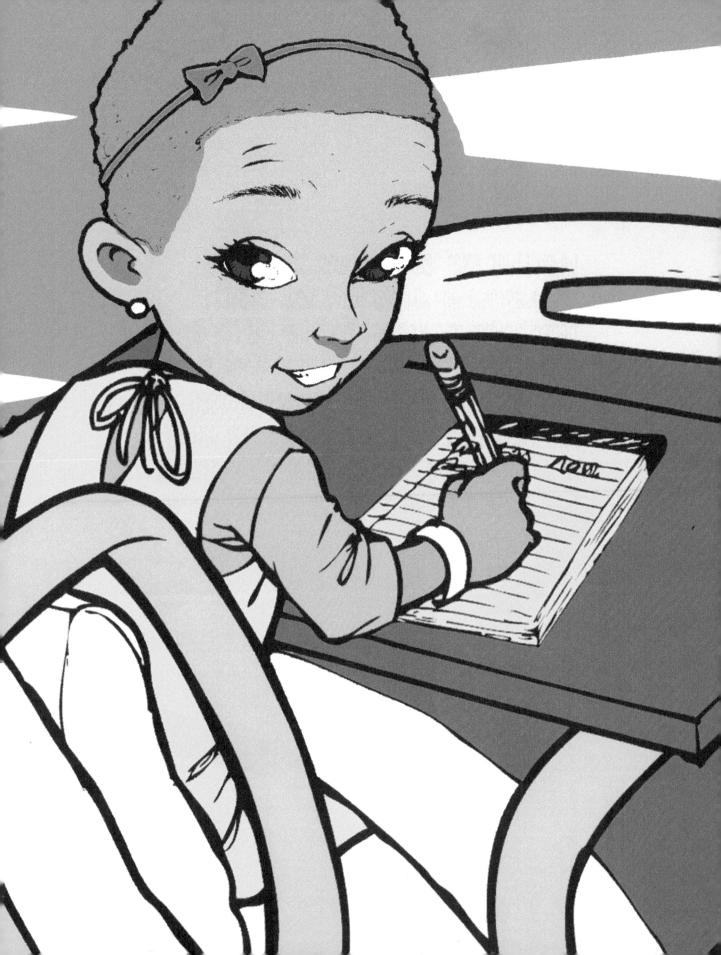

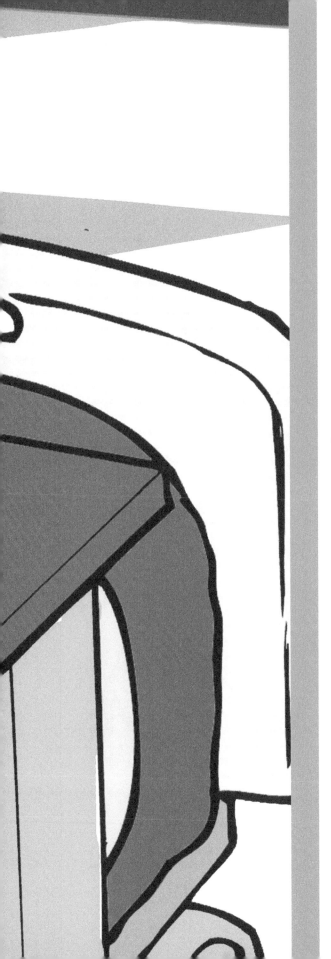

This is me in the hospital waiting to see my doctor. I'm sure you're wondering why I'm writing this story from the hospital.

Keep reading so I can tell you about it!

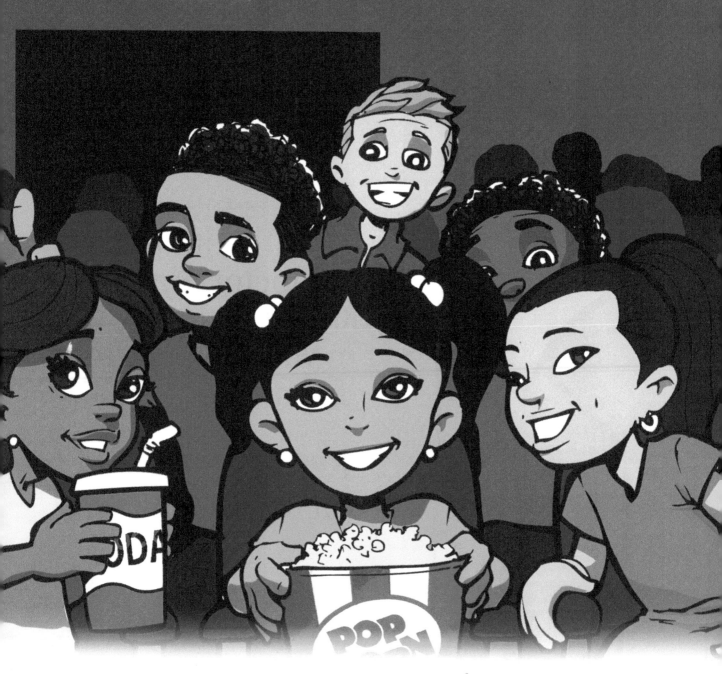

Before I started coming to the
hospital everyday, I used to enjoy doing
regular kid things like going
to the movies with my friends.

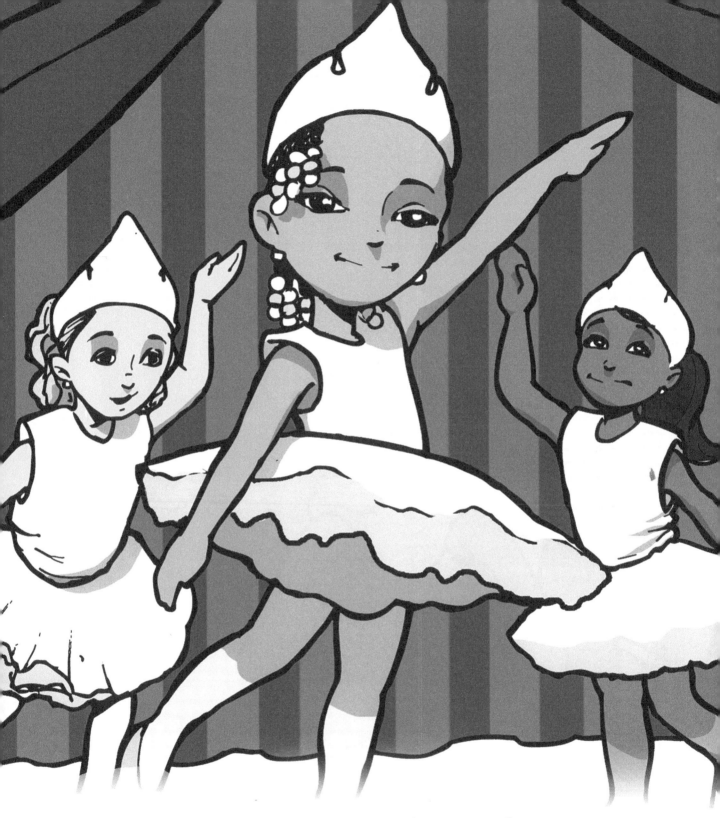

My favorite day of the week was
Wednesday because I had dance
class after school and I love to dance!

On the day of my first dance recital, I had a tummy ache and started feeling very tired.

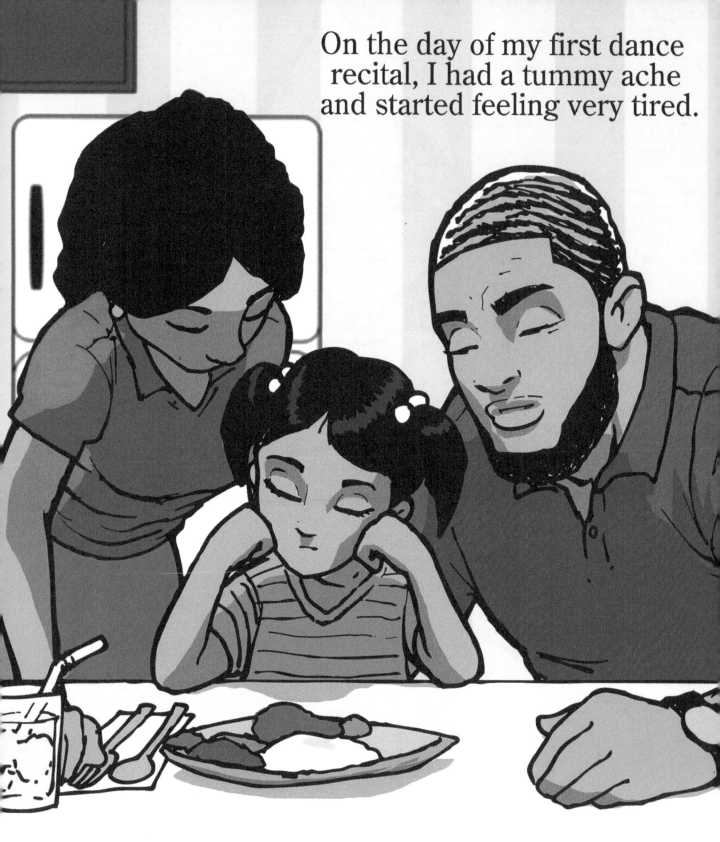

My parents kept trying to get me to eat but I didn't want to eat anything.

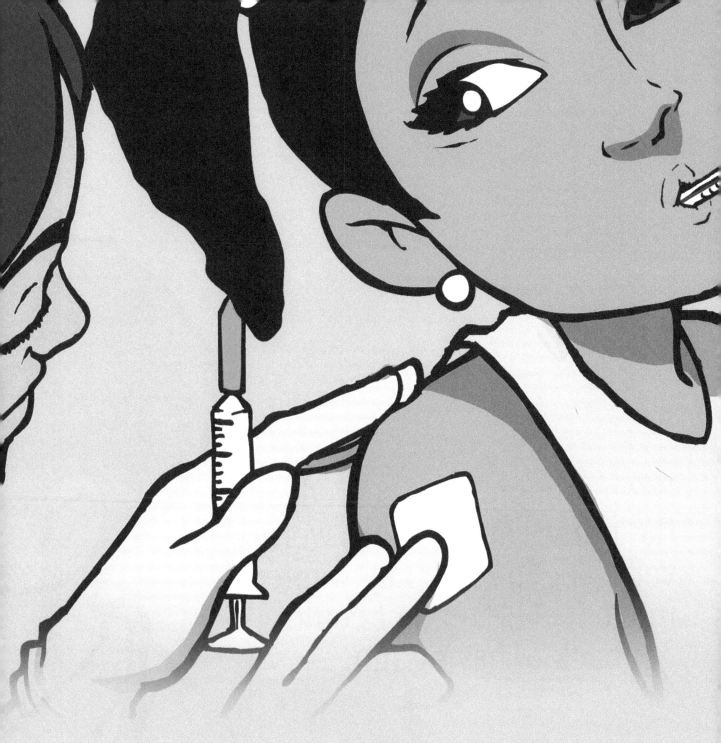

My mom said my forehead felt warm so my parents took me to the hospital to see a doctor. I've always been afraid of hospitals because I'm afraid of all the needles. They feel like somebody is pinching you!

Even though I was scared, all the nurses and doctors were very nice to me. They wanted me to feel better so I could get back to having fun.

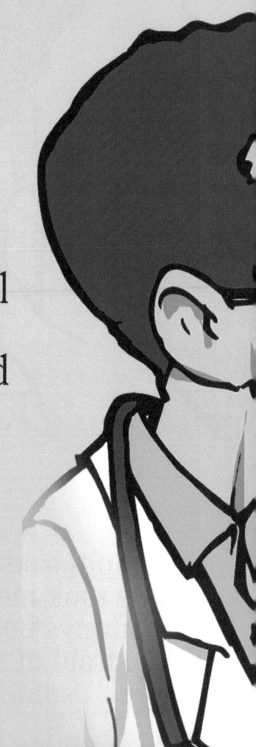

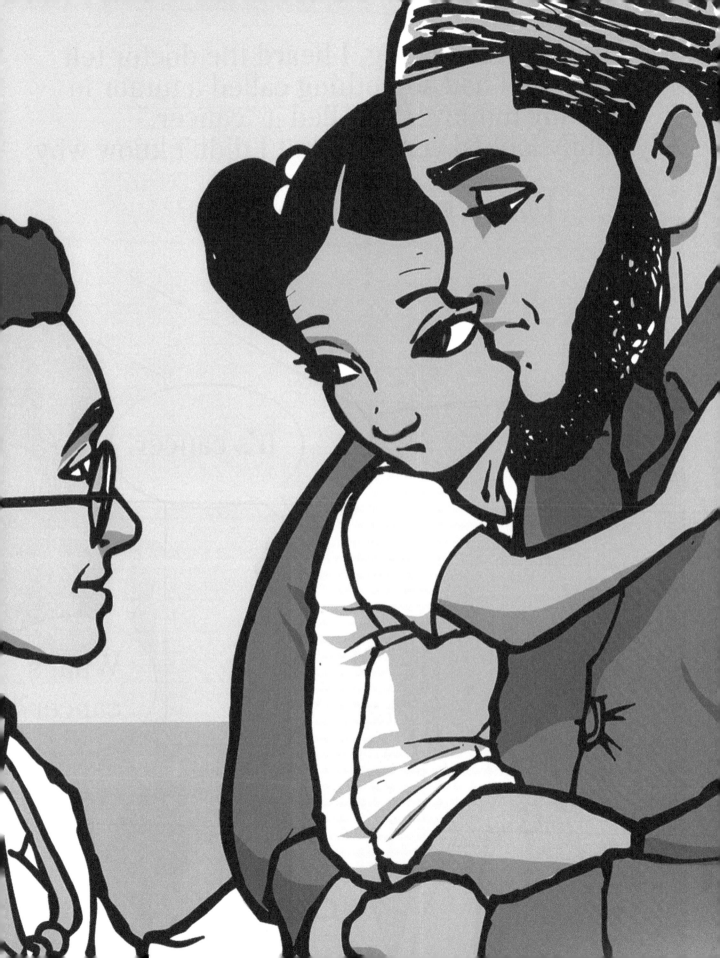

After all of the testing, I heard the doctor tell my family I had something called a tumor in my tummy. He called it "cancer."
My family looked very sad, but I didn't know why.

Do you know what cancer is?

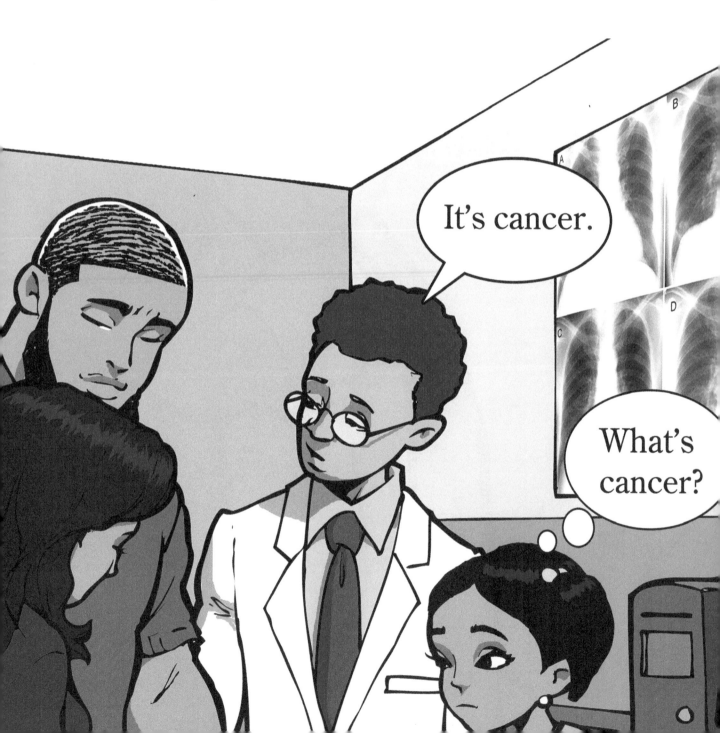

They told me cancer is a bad
disease that would hurt my body.

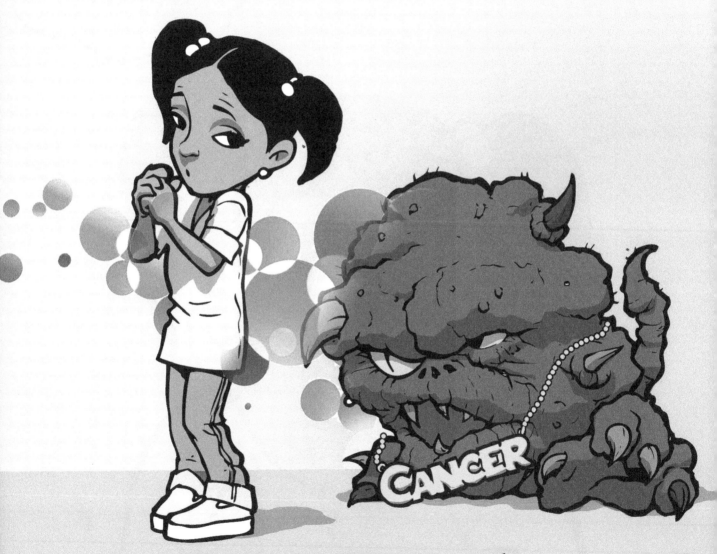

It meant I would have to go to the
hospital a lot and I couldn't go
to school or dance class anymore.

When I heard this, I was very sad.

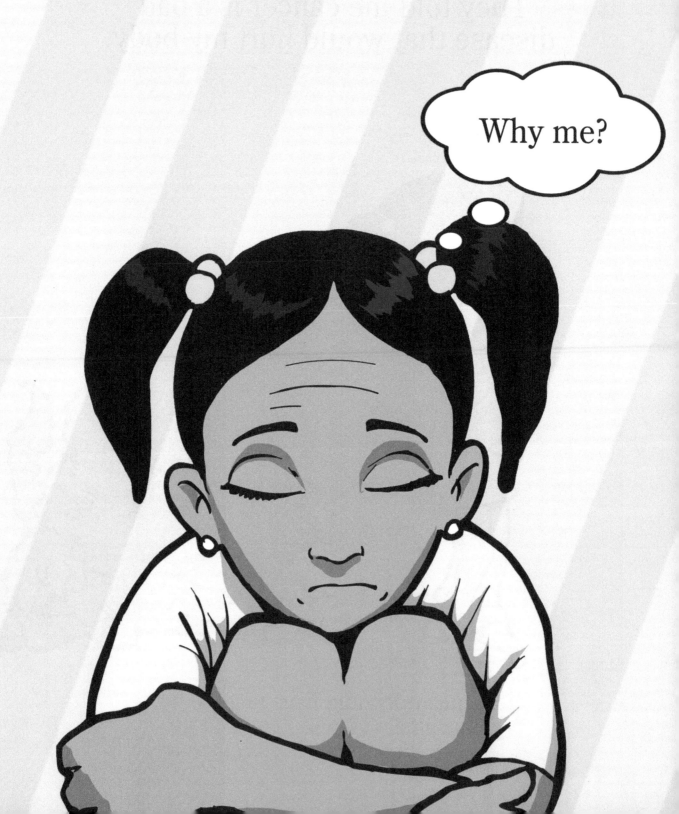

But my parents told me, "stay strong."

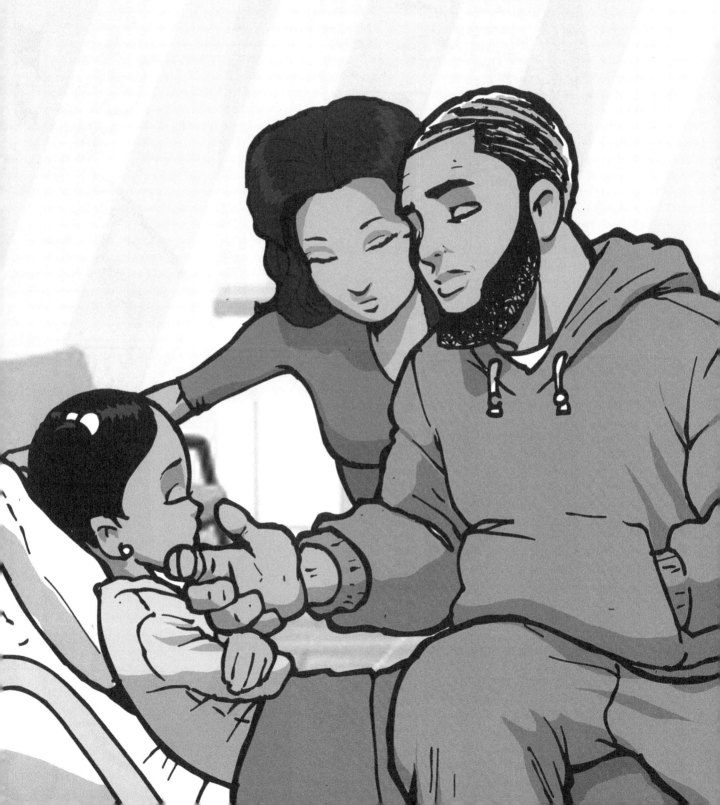

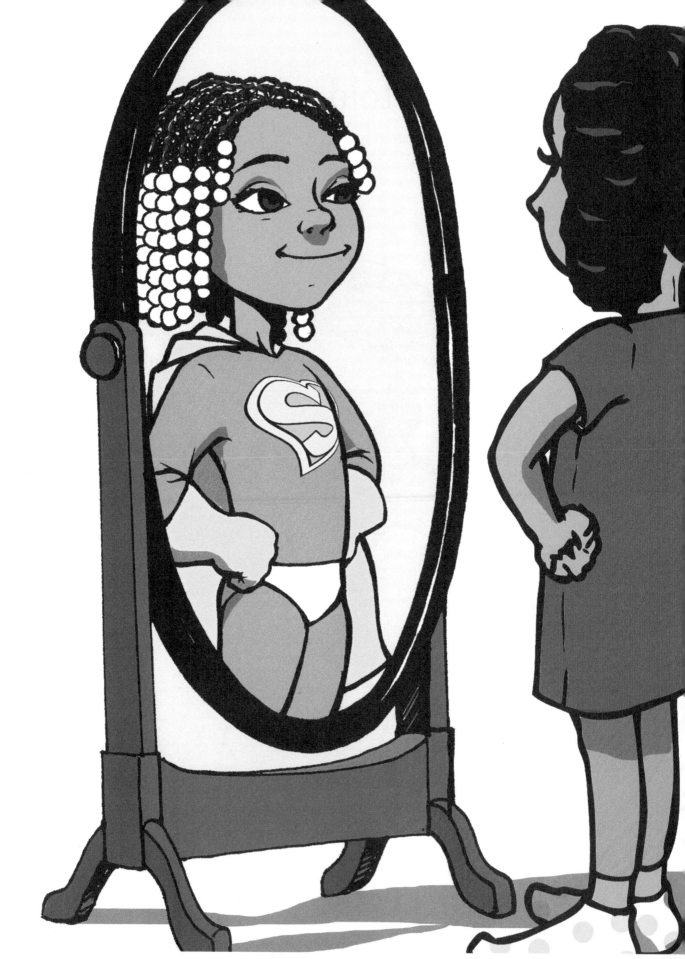

So I did!

Then my doctor said, "We can try chemotherapy."

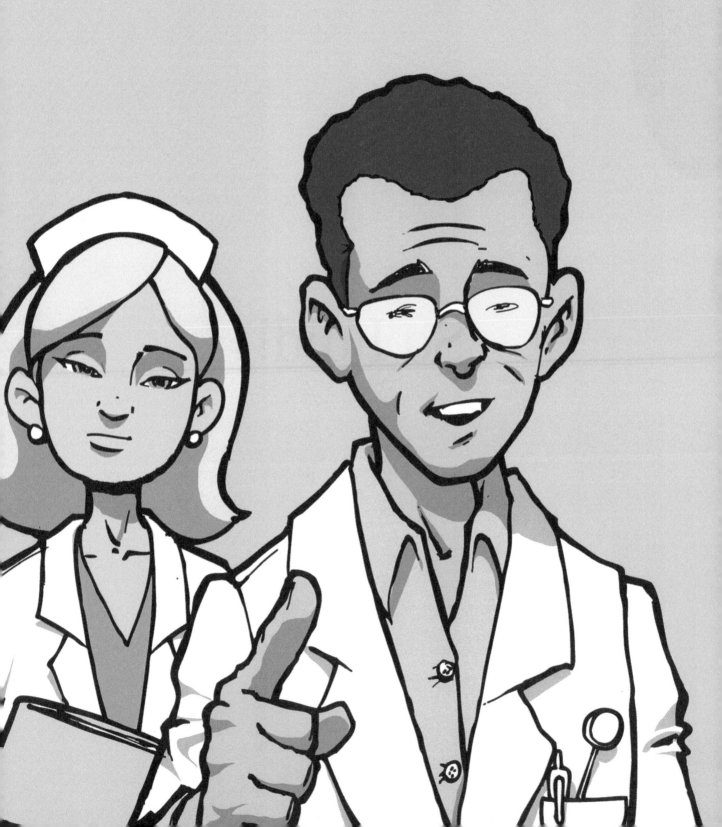

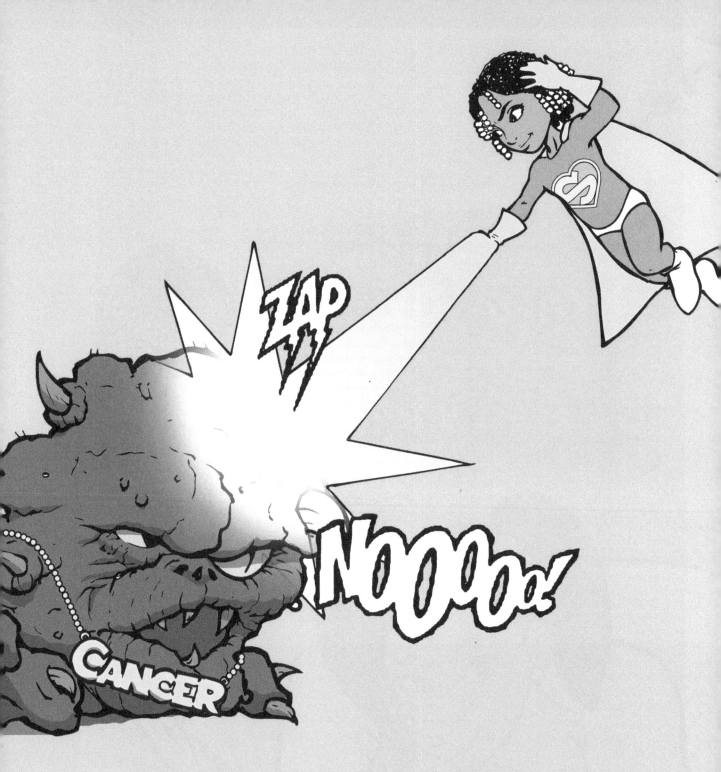

Che-mo-therapy is the medicine
that helps my body beat up cancer
by shrinking the tumor. They call it
chemo for short.

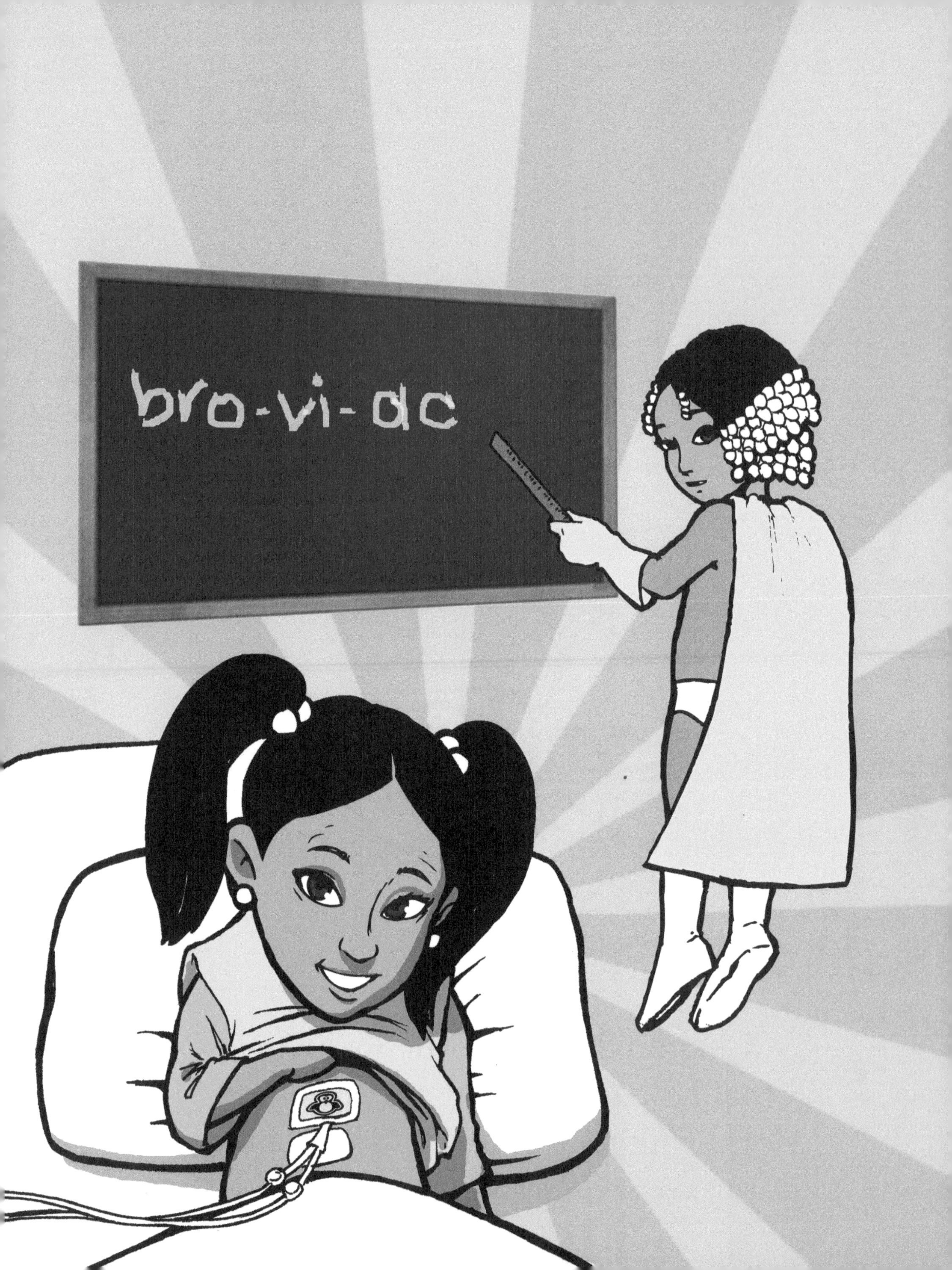
bro-vi-ac

When getting chemo, doctors put tubes in your chest so you don't have to get a bunch of needles poked in you. There are two kinds of tubes: a bro-vi-ac and a port.

My doctor gave me the broviac catheter.

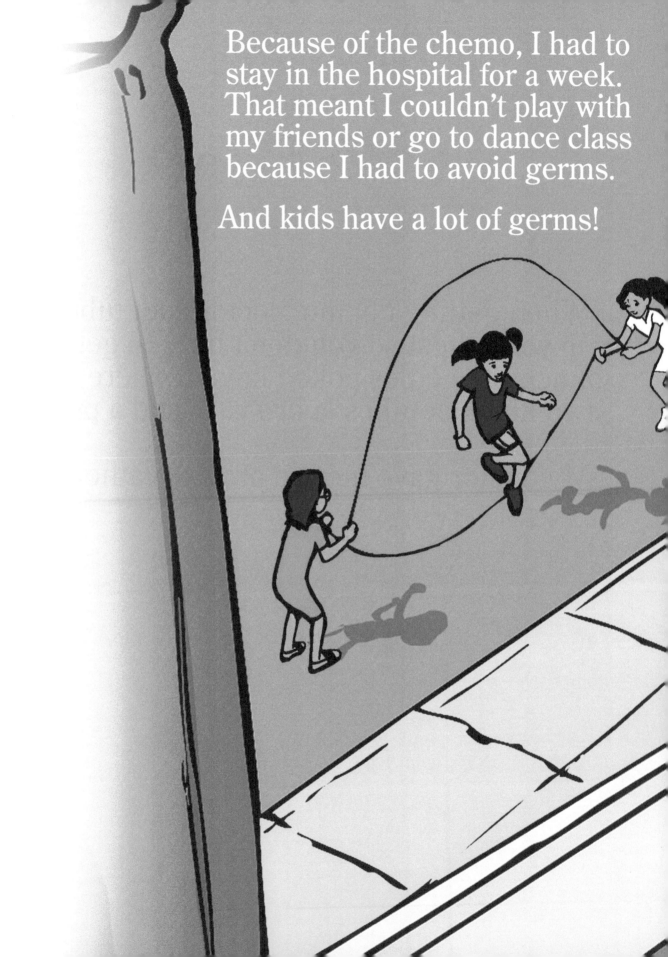

Because of the chemo, I had to stay in the hospital for a week. That meant I couldn't play with my friends or go to dance class because I had to avoid germs.

And kids have a lot of germs!

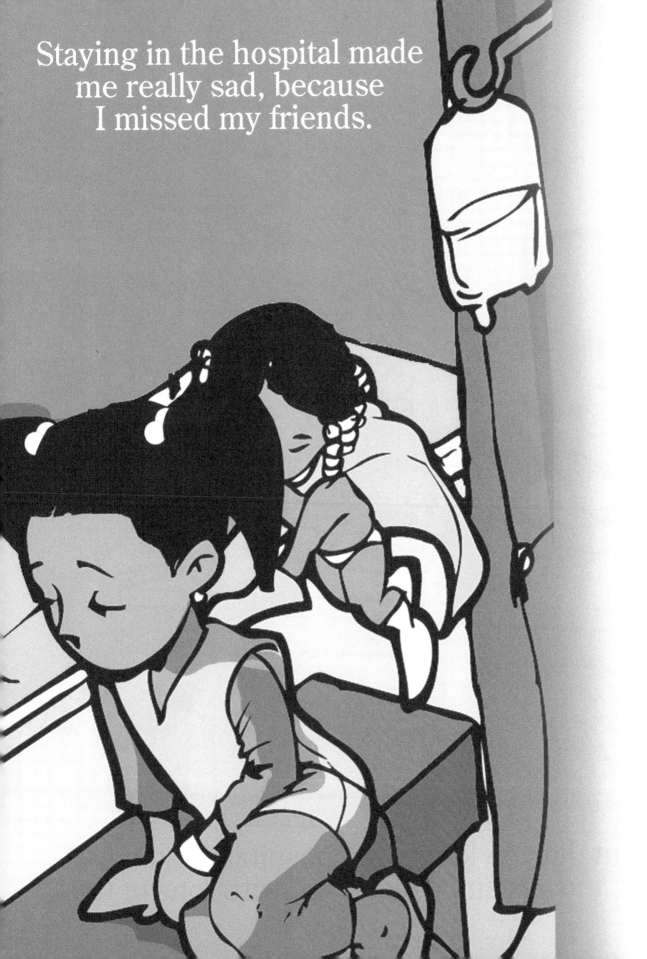

Staying in the hospital made
me really sad, because
I missed my friends.

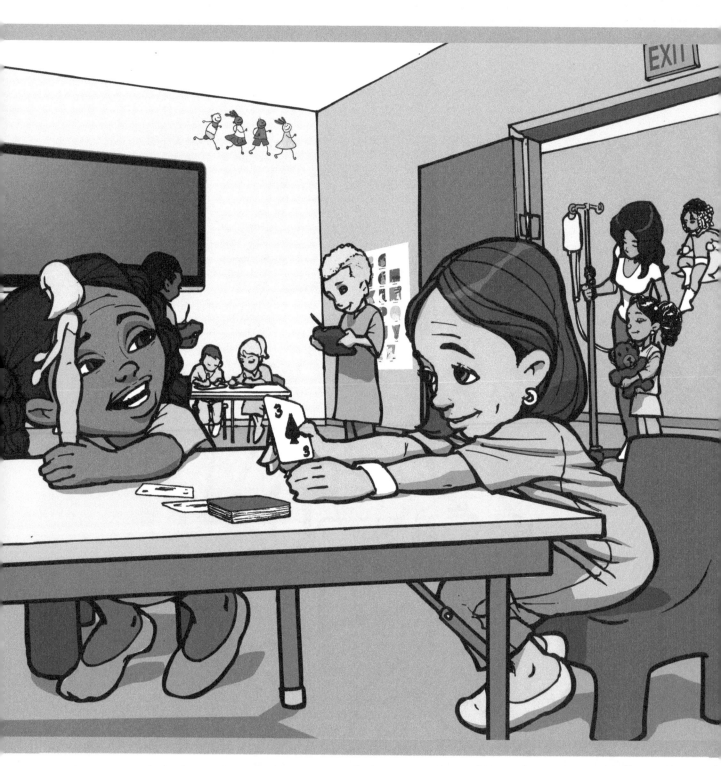

But did you know that hospitals also have
TVs, movies and a playroom with tons of toys?

...And great food! My favorite is the cheese steak.

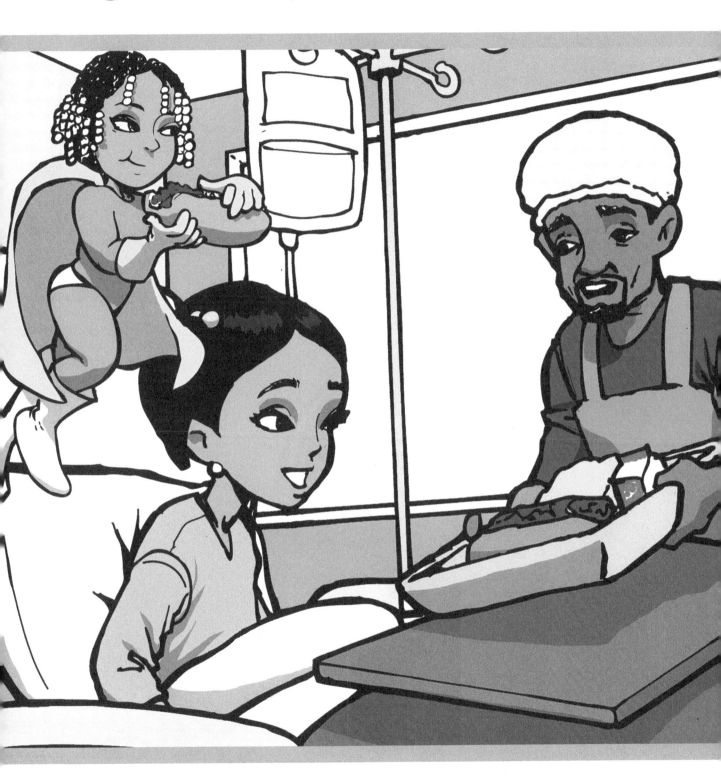

What's your favorite food?

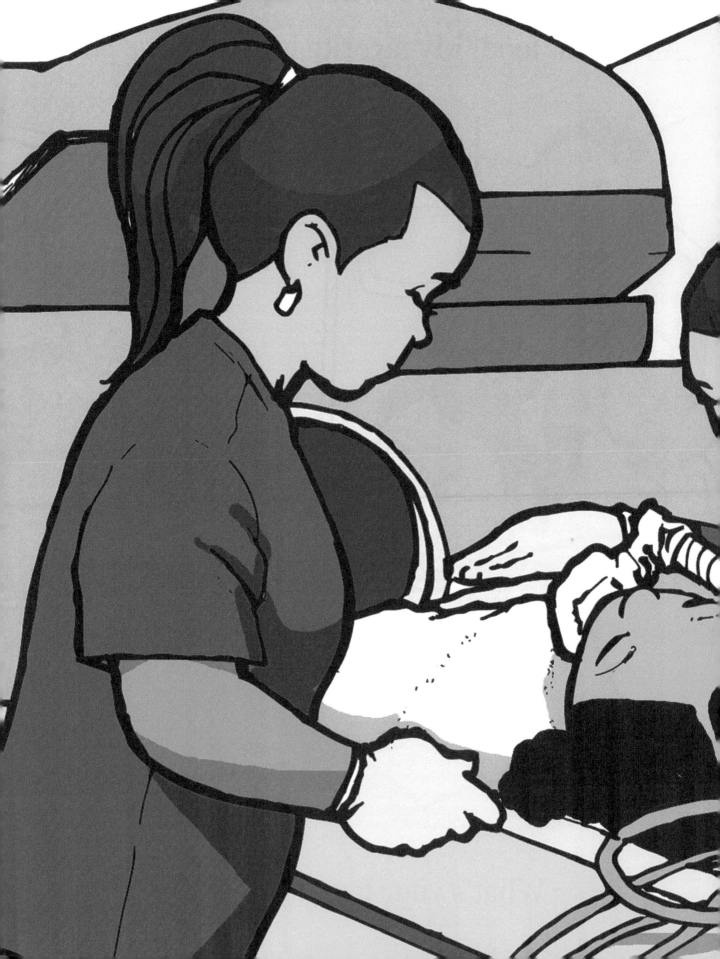

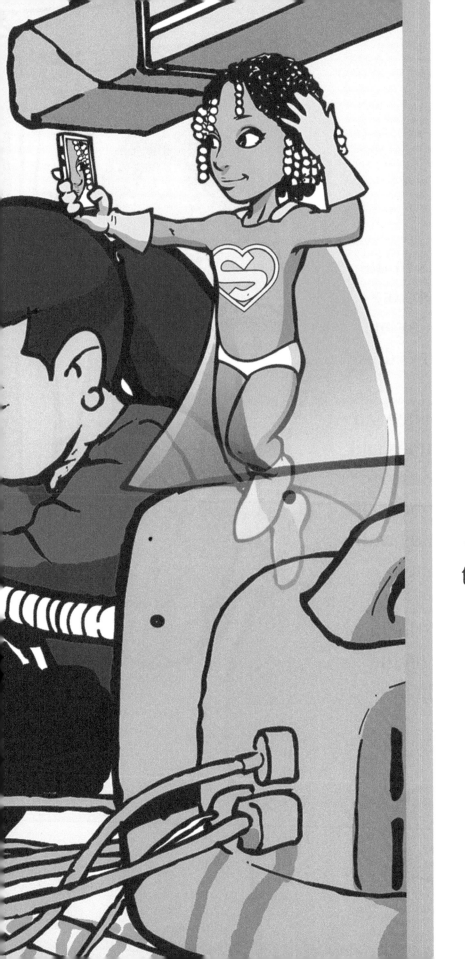

During the day, I sat underneath really big machines for MRIs, CT scans and X-rays. I don't remember what the words mean but the tests helped the doctor take pictures of the inside of my body... Like a camera!

I had to spend some nights in the hospital connected to more big machines with tubes sticking out of me, which meant more needles!

But the nurses were nice. They put dog stickers on top of the tubes and made it look like a dog house to keep me from pulling the tubes out. They also gave me Band-Aids with cartoon characters on them.

Plus, the machines told the doctors what my body was doing on the inside so they could help me.

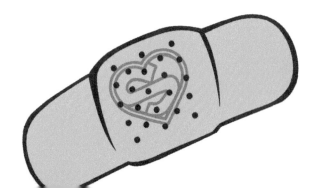

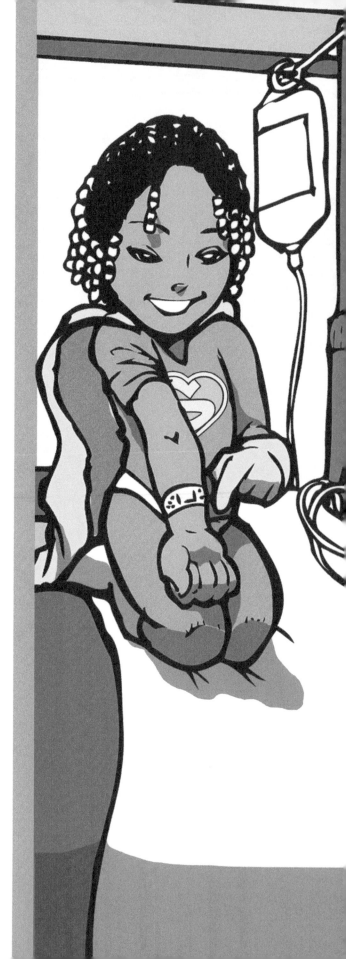

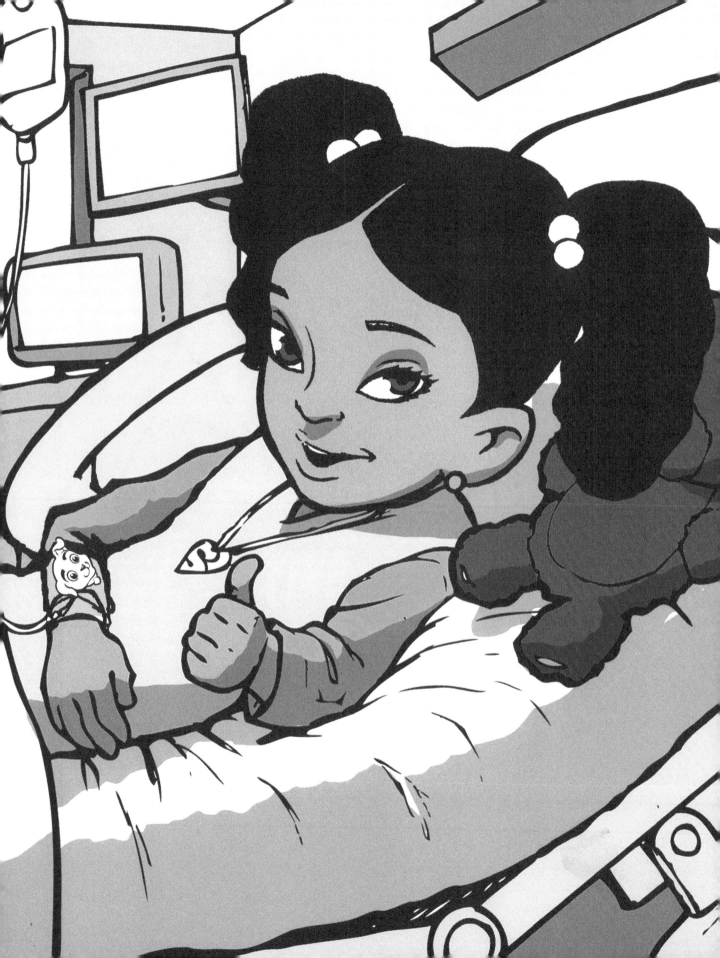

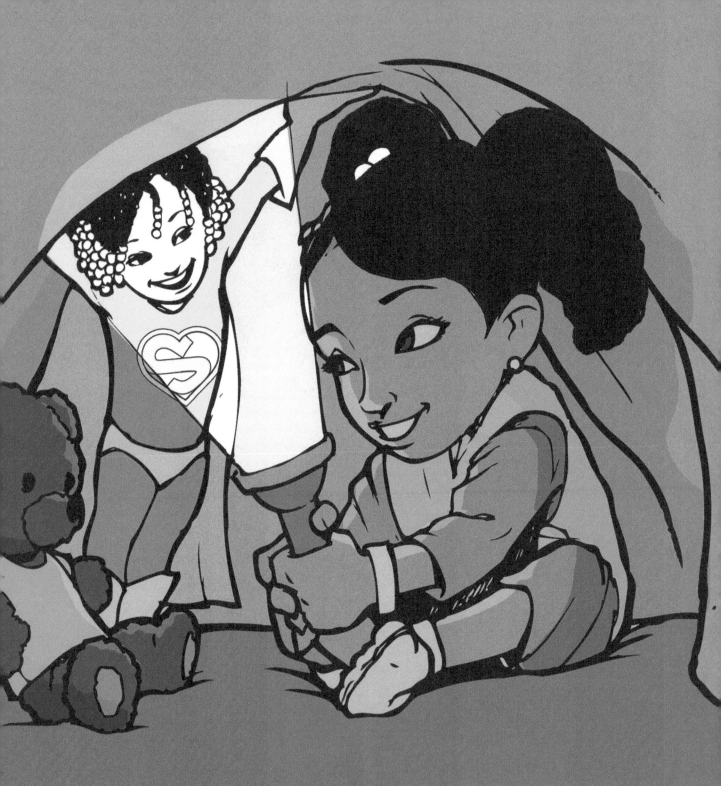

It was scary at night when the lights went out.

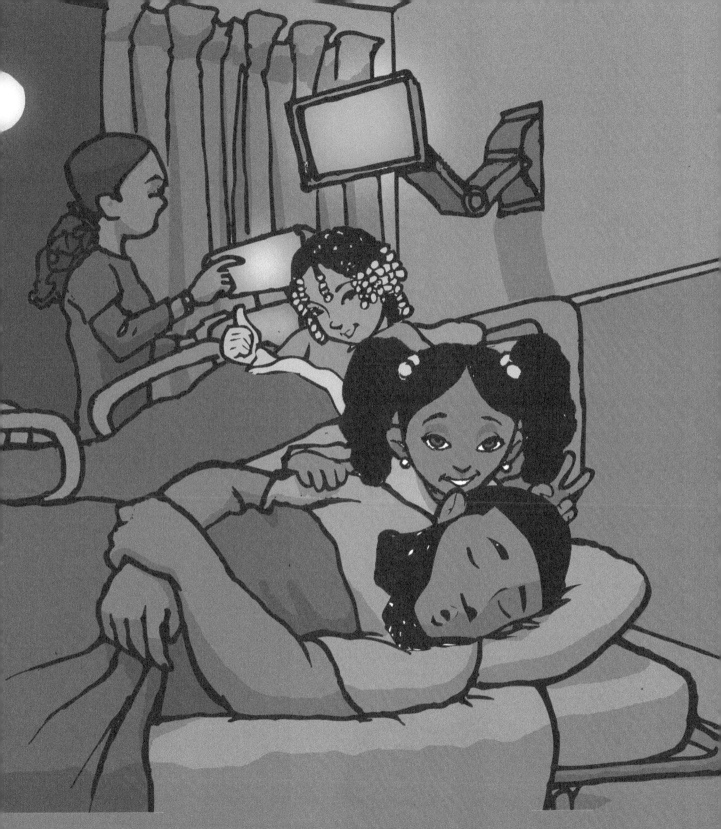

But the hospital let my family spend the night with me. And even if my family couldn't be there, I knew I was never alone.

Because I was Still Strong.

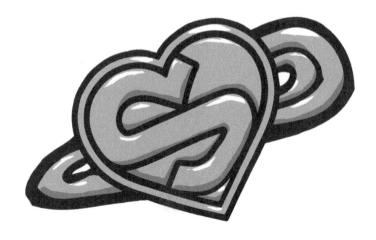

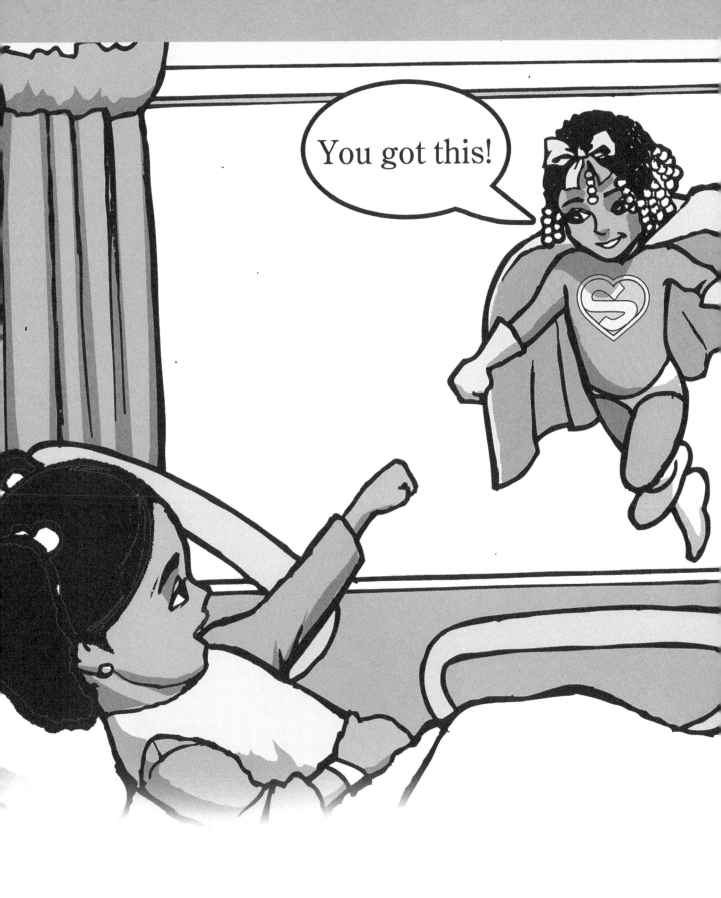

With my chemo treatments, there were good days and there were bad days.

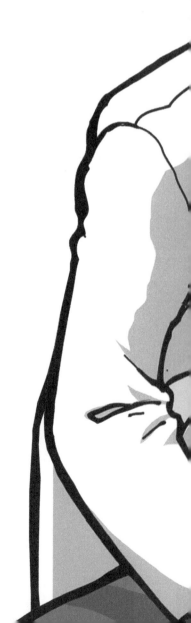

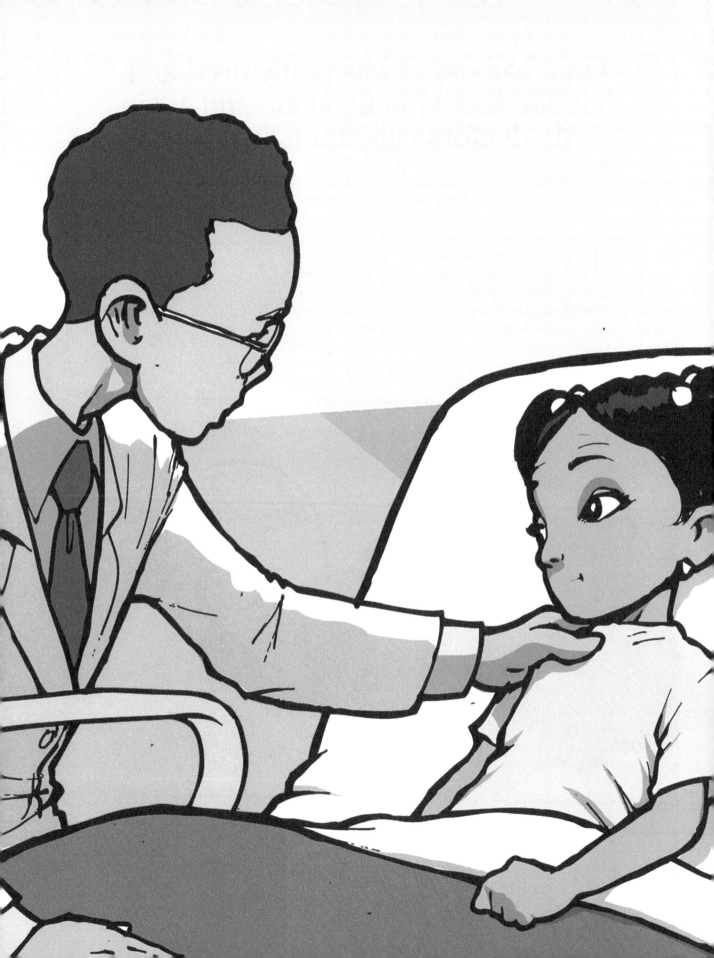

On a bad day, I was really tired and
felt like throwing up again and again.
My doctors called this nau-se-a.

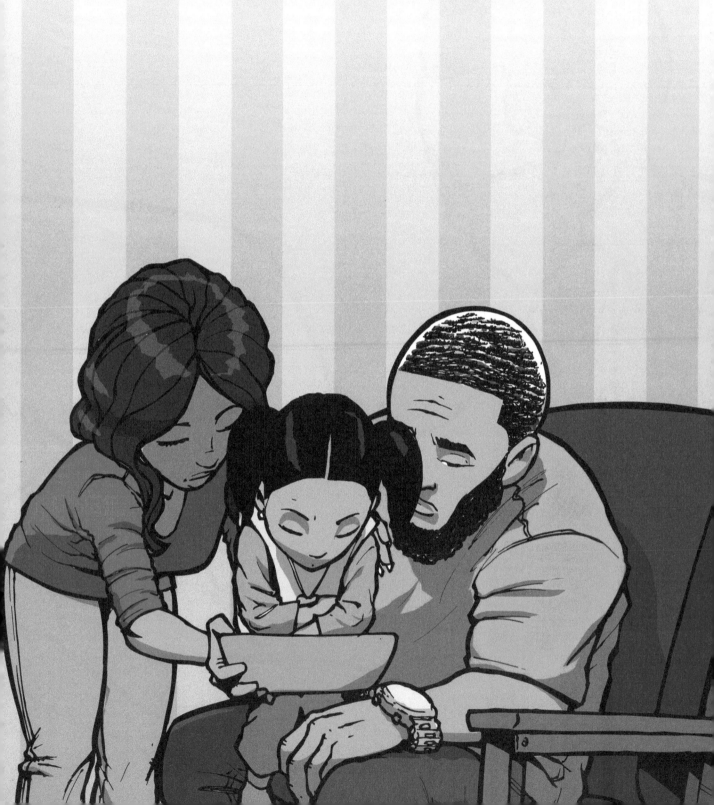

So the doctors gave me this cool tube in my nose that allowed me to get all of my nutrition so I can keep my big strong muscles to beat up cancer. They even let me put a penguin on there. I named him Ice Cream. LOL!

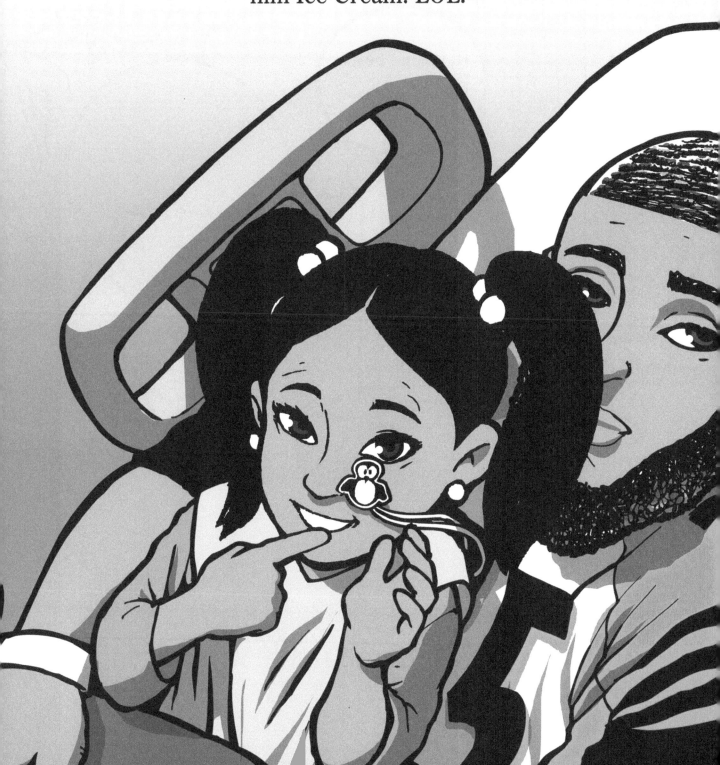

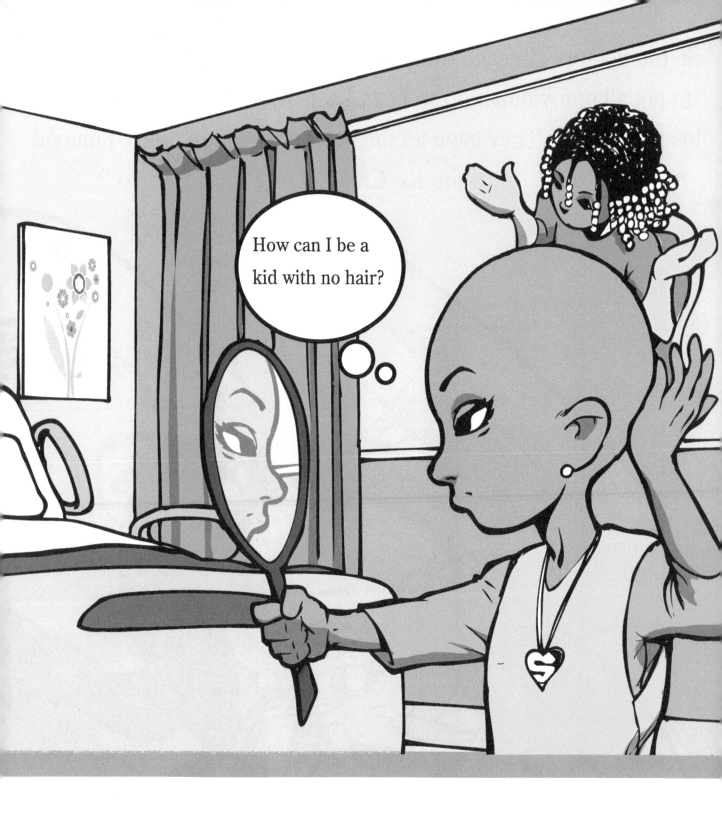

Unfortunately, the chemo made my hair fall out.

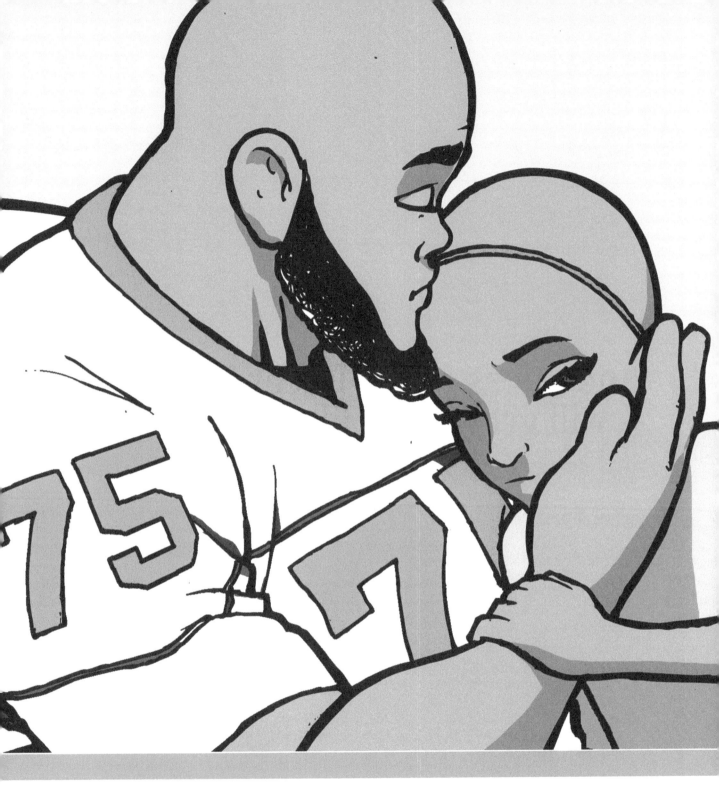

But my dad told me, "Beauty comes from the inside. With or without your hair, you are beautiful. Stay strong."

And guess what? I heard my hair will grow back like Rapunzel!

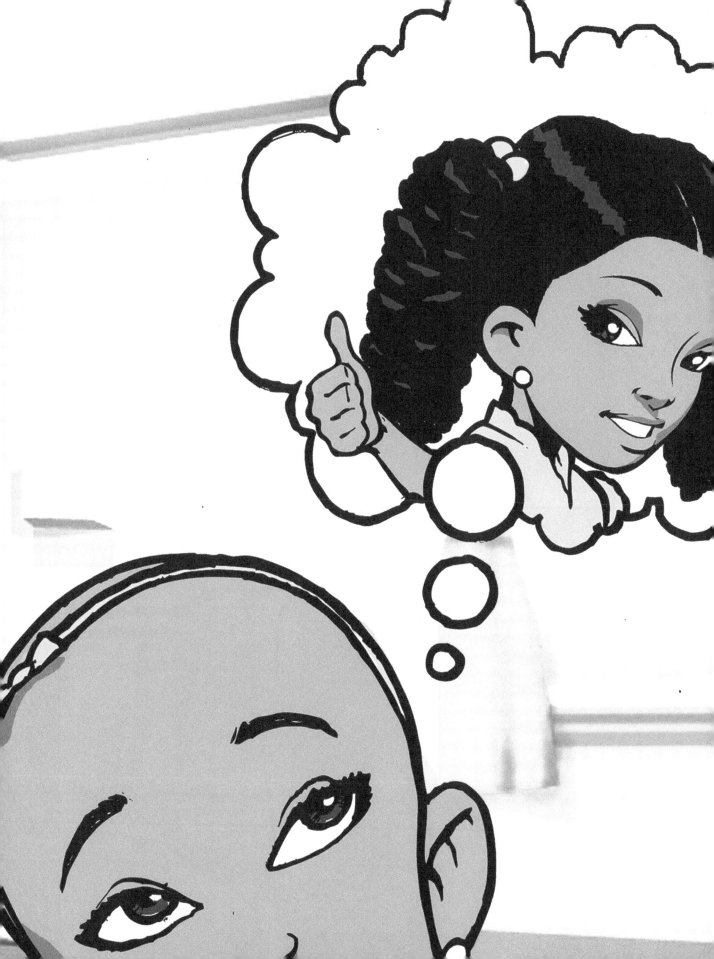

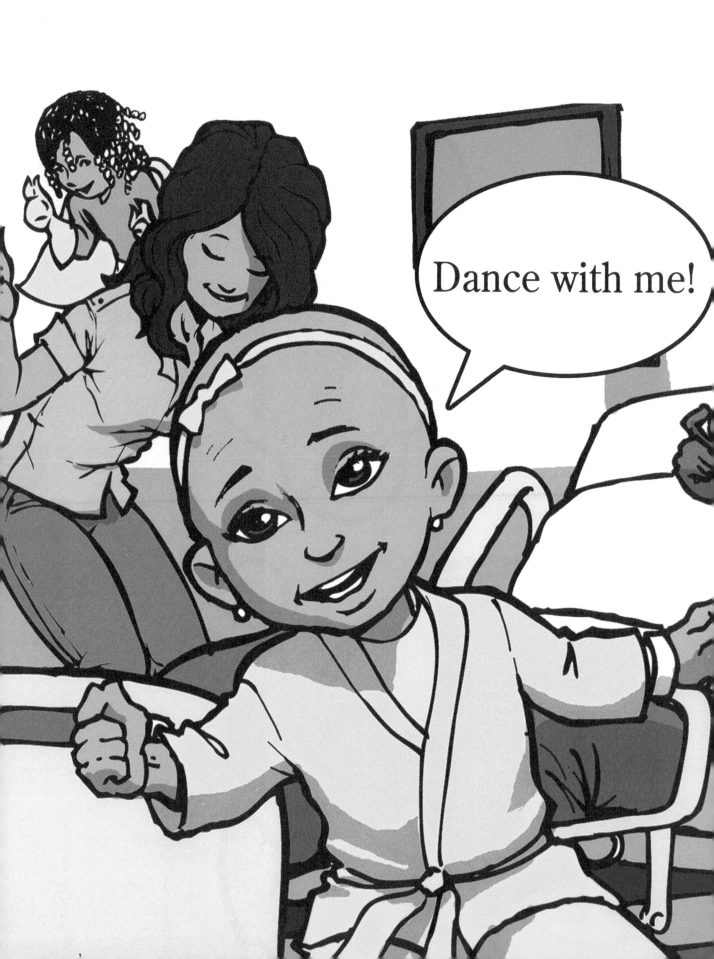

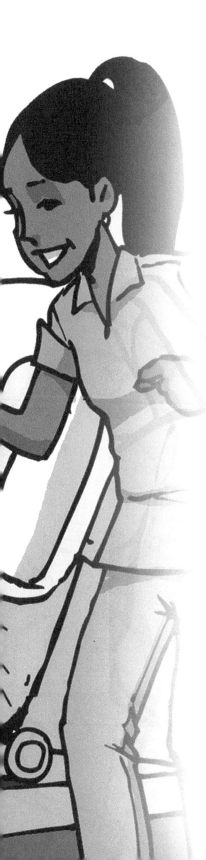

On a good day, I felt great and I felt like dancing.

The chemo treatments helped shrink the cancer so my doctor could work on my tummy and get the cancer out.

The doctors called it surgery. Surgery meant the doctor had to make a small cut to get inside my tummy.

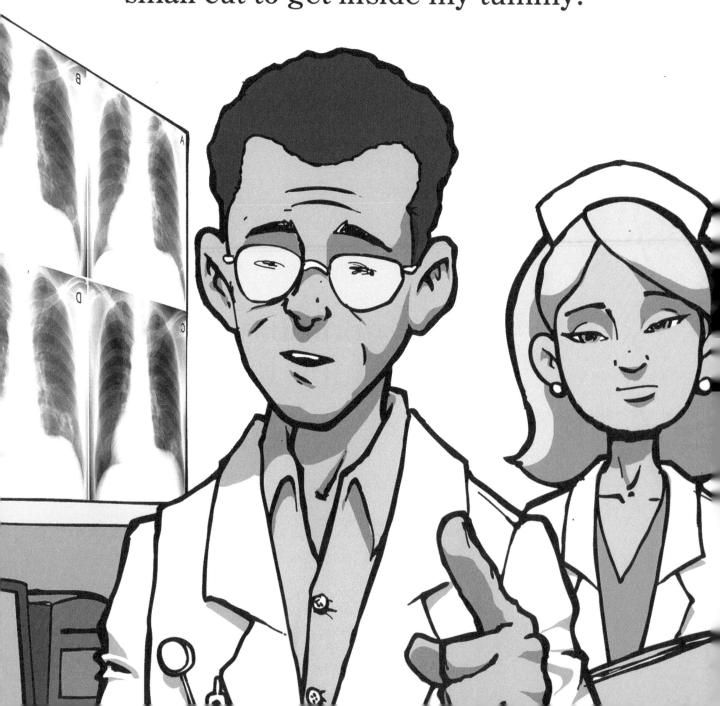

"Like a paper cut?" I asked.

"No, a little bigger than that," my doctor said.

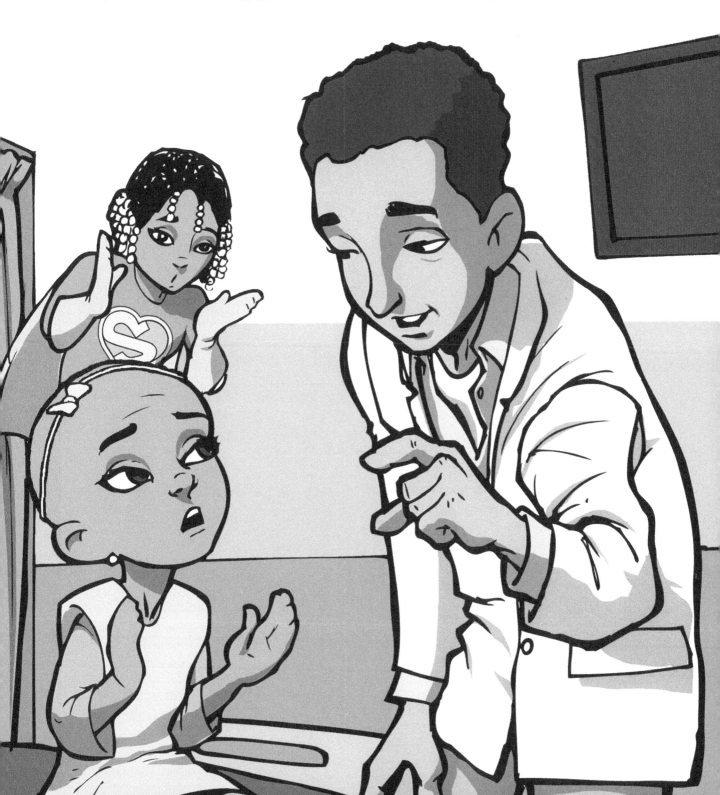

Aaaa

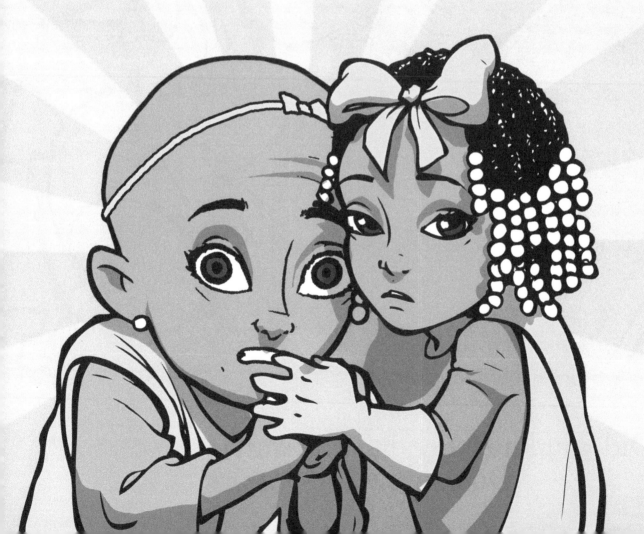

On the day of my surgery, my dad told me when it was all over I'd have a scar like a warrior and could show everyone my scar to let them know I was Leah Strong and I beat cancer.

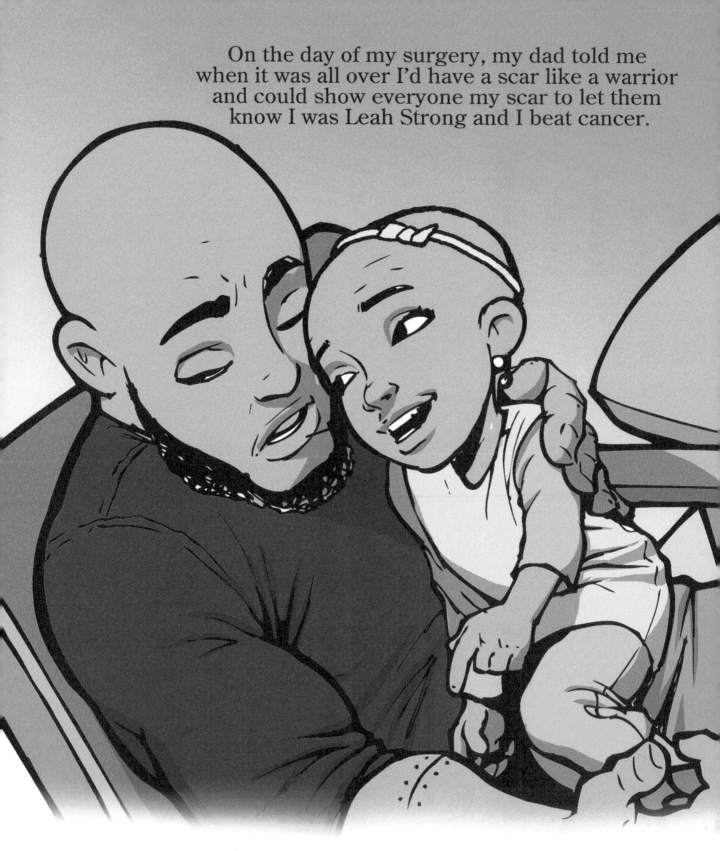

Did you know my dad has warrior scars too?
Do you have any scars?

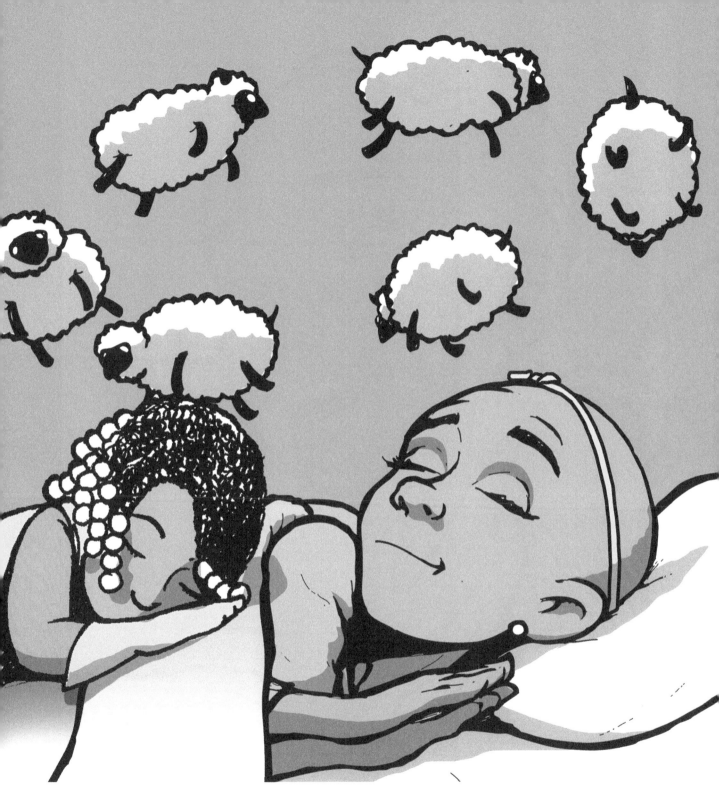

Right before the surgery, the doctor gave me medicine that made me laugh a lot and also very sleepy, so I wouldn't even feel it.

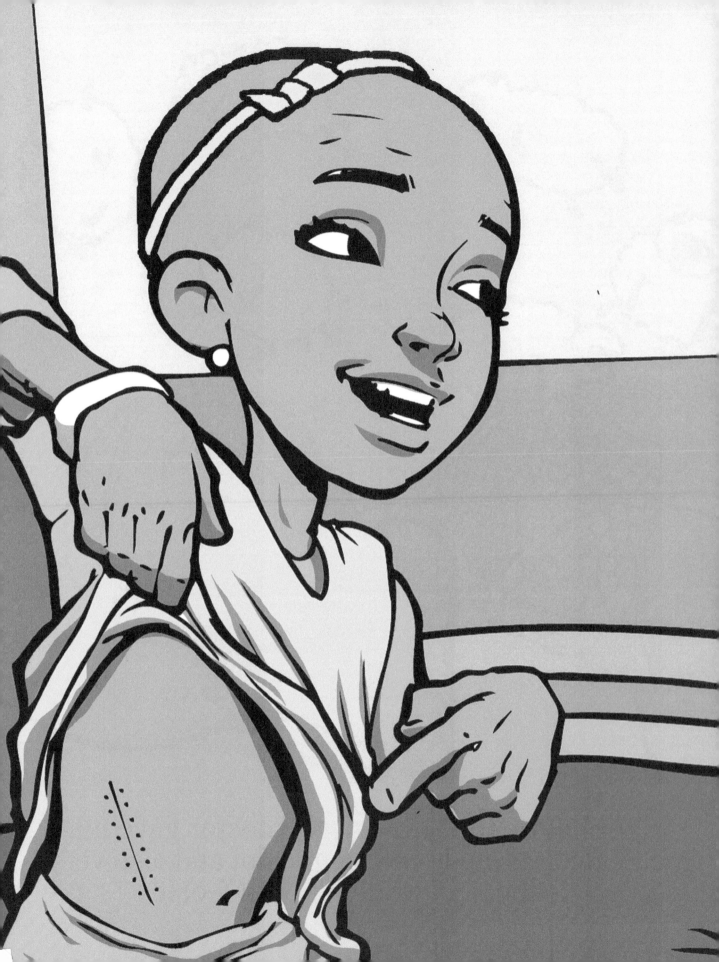

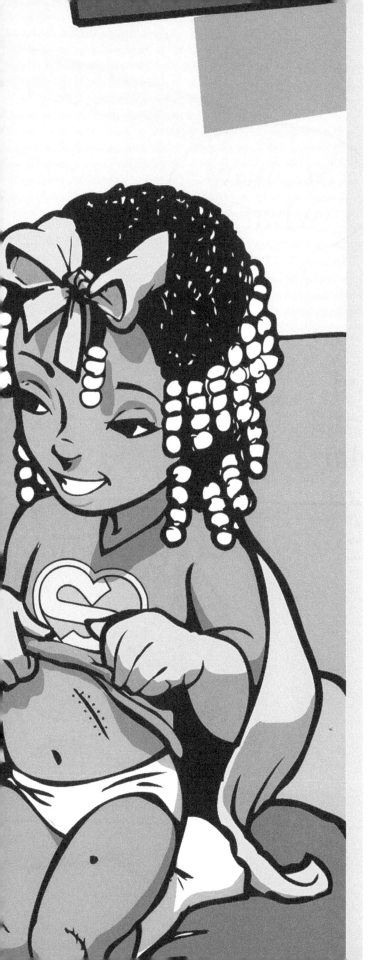

When I woke up,
the surgery was over.

It wasn't as bad as I
thought it would be.

And look, my scar
isn't that bad either!

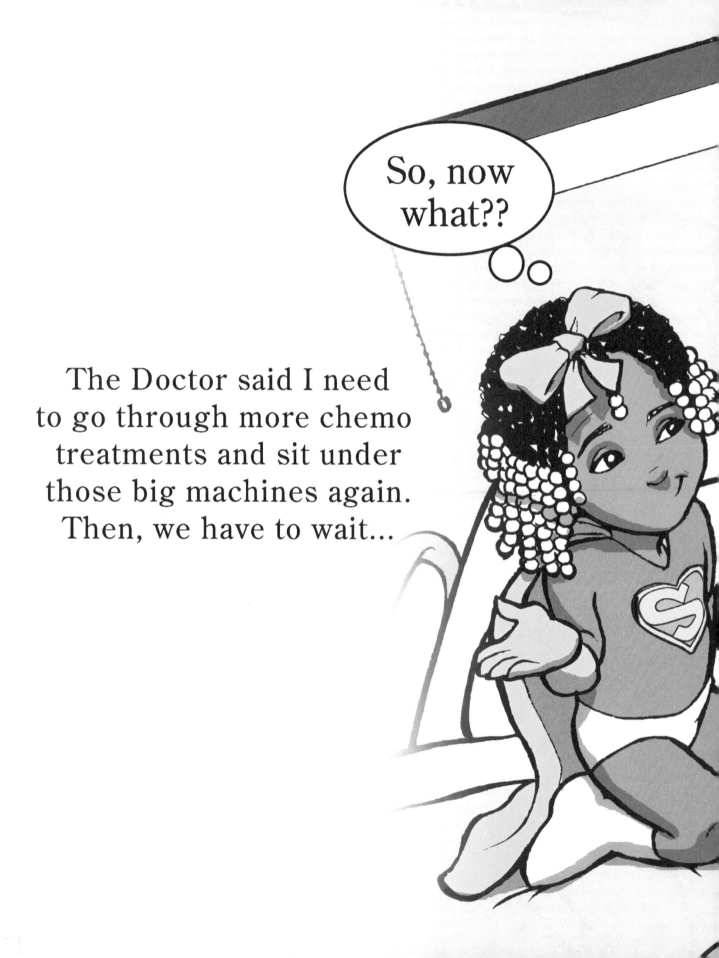

So, now what??

The Doctor said I need to go through more chemo treatments and sit under those big machines again. Then, we have to wait...

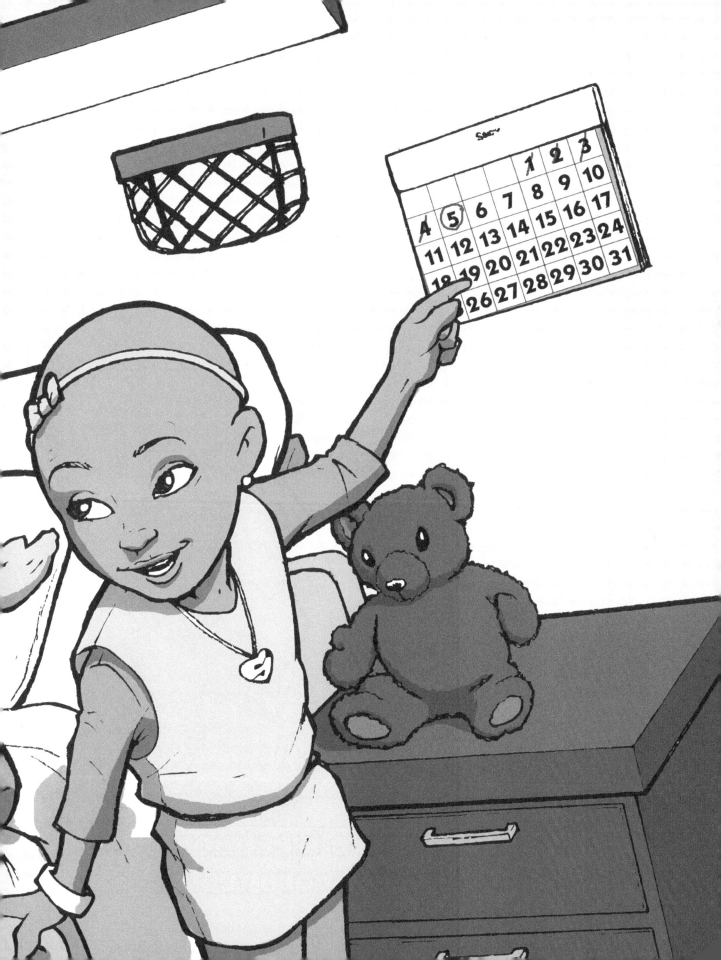

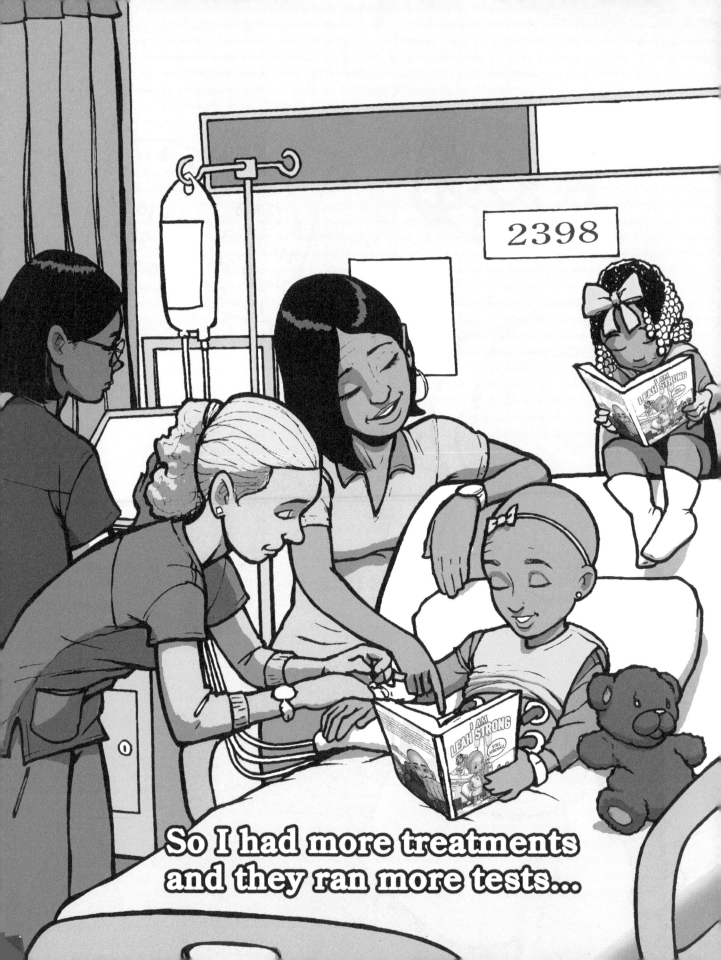

So I had more treatments
and they ran more tests...

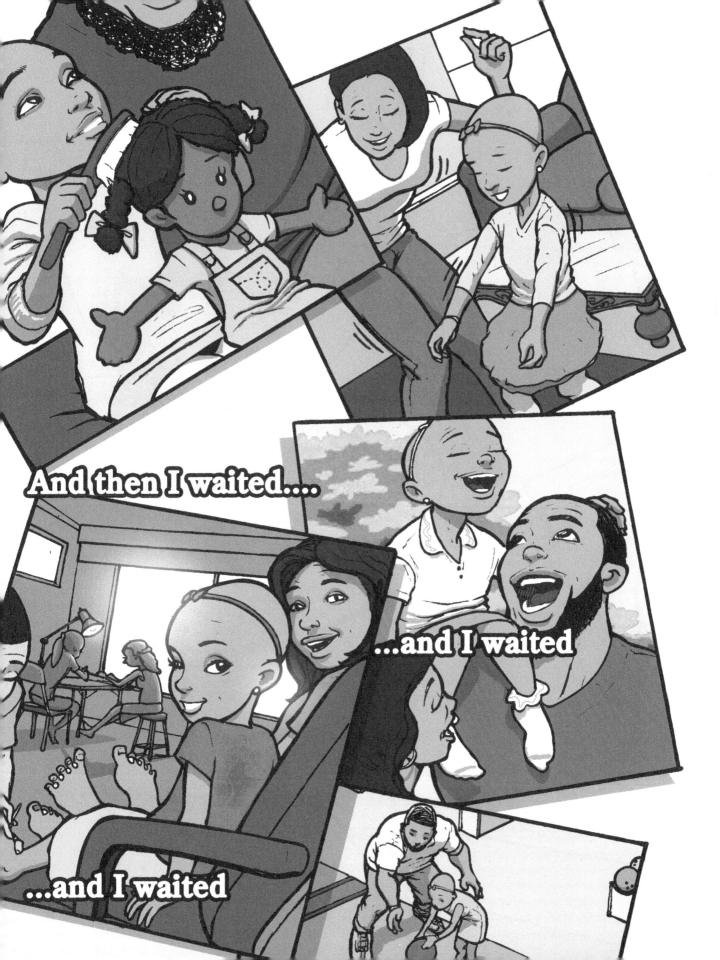

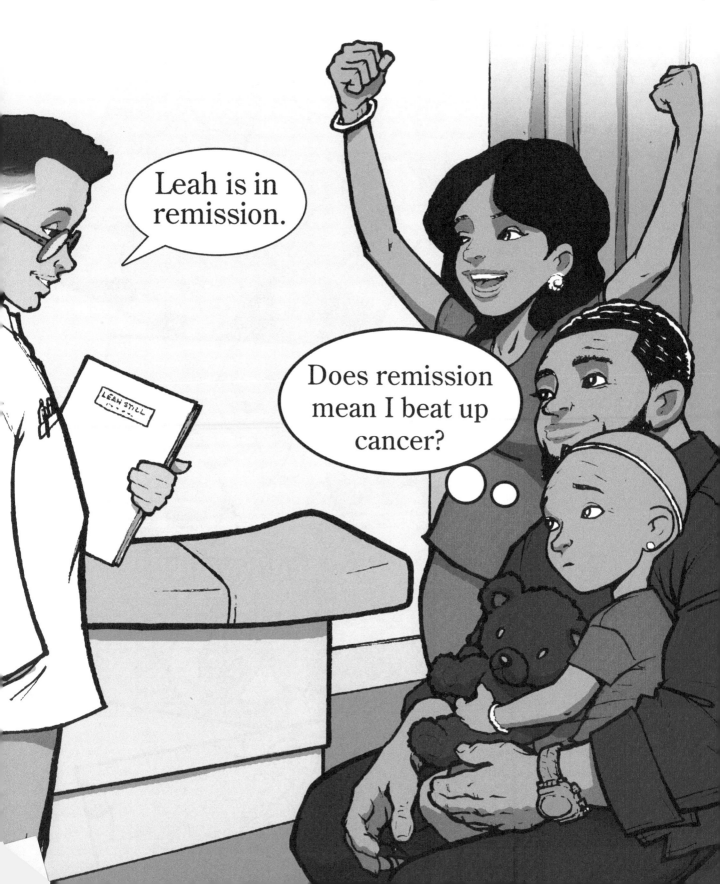

My parents said remission means
I fought so hard that the
Cancer got scared and ran away!

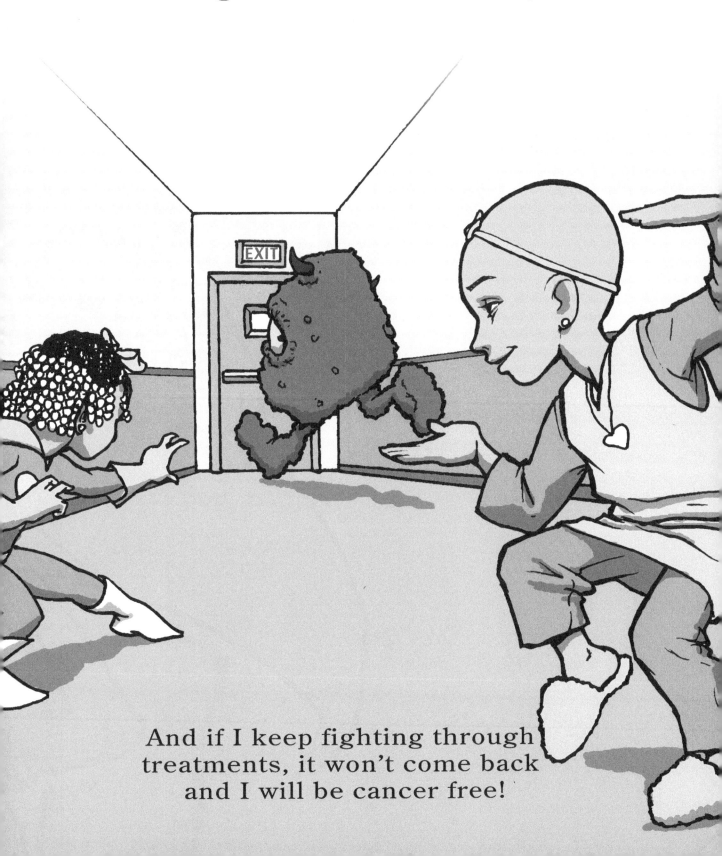

And if I keep fighting through
treatments, it won't come back
and I will be cancer free!

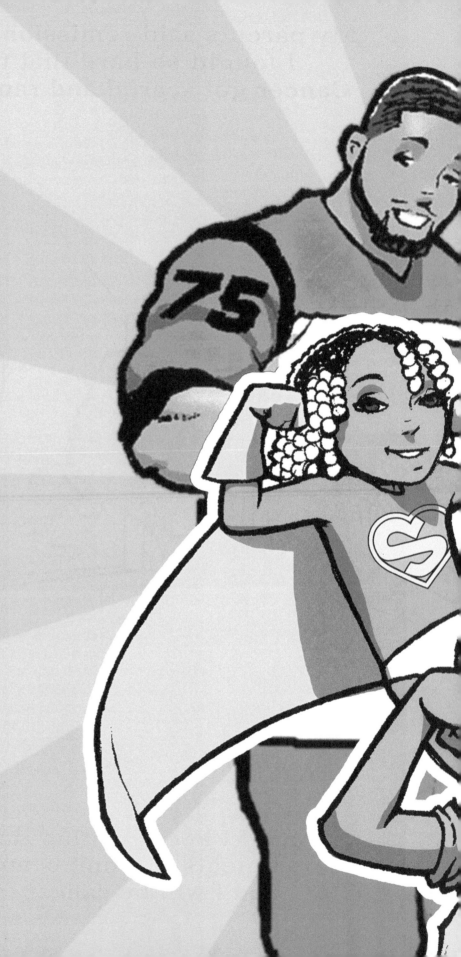

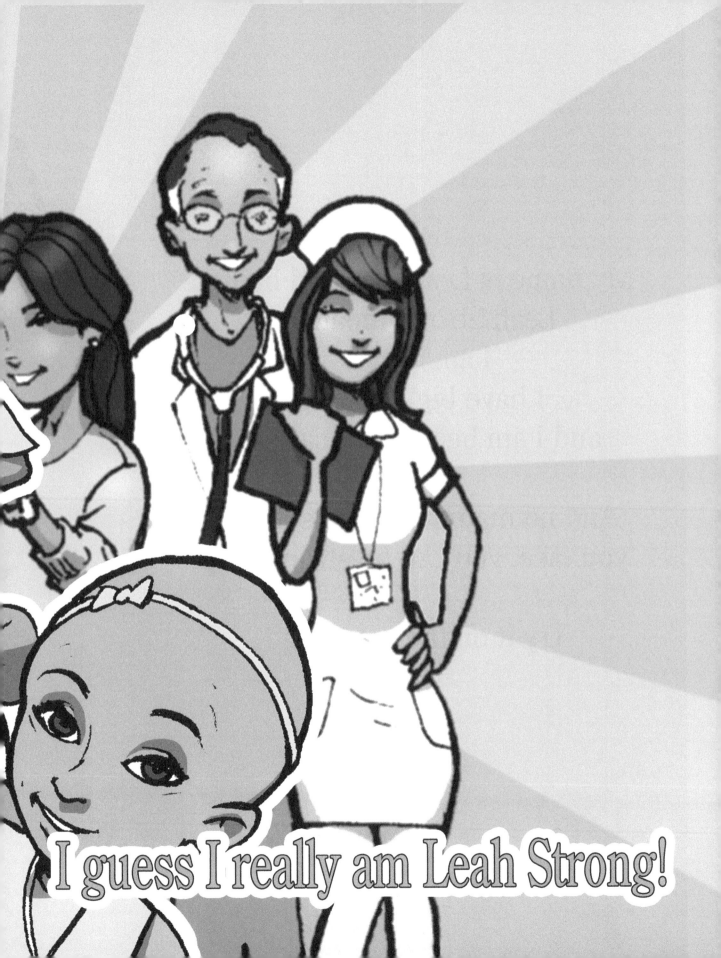

My name is Leah Still and being
Leah Strong means...
I am brave.
I have big muscles
and I am beating up cancer.

And no matter what obstacles
you face, you can be strong too!

Try it on the next page

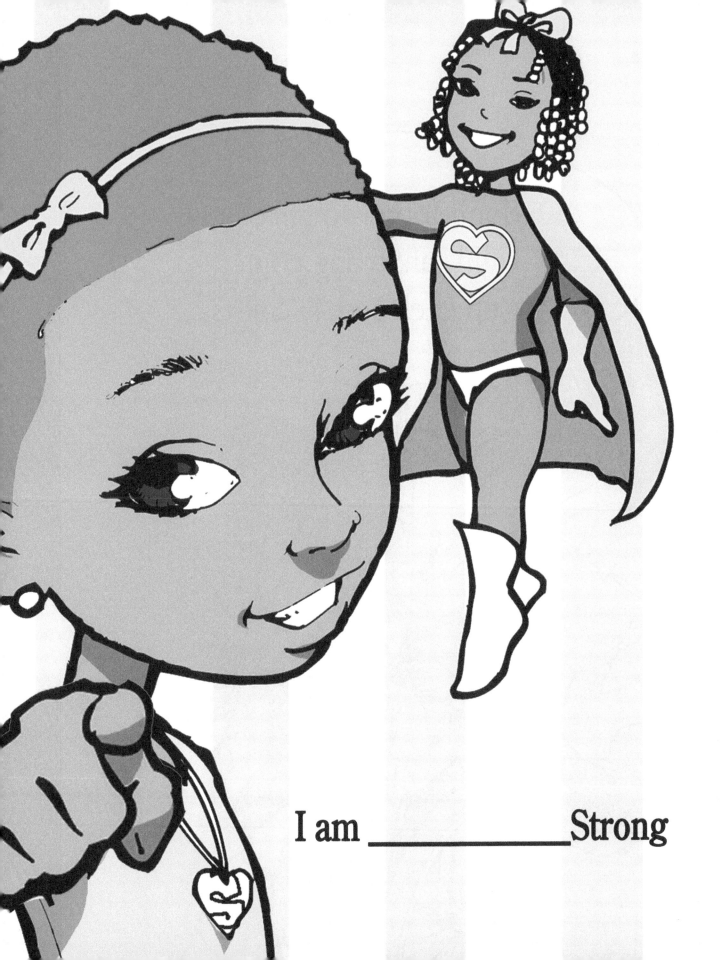

I am _____ Strong

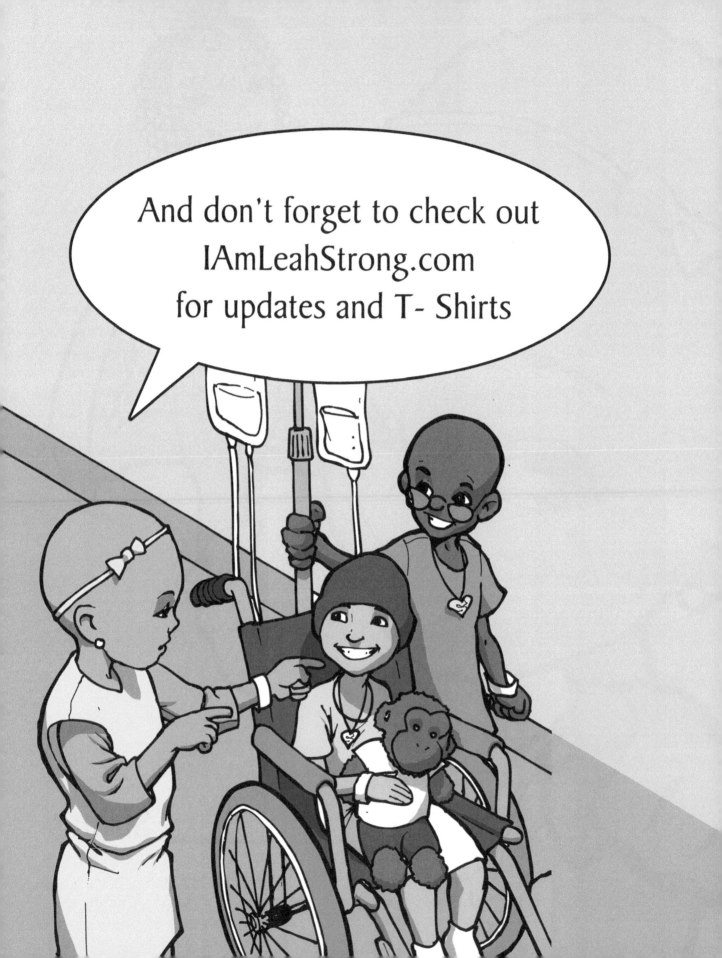

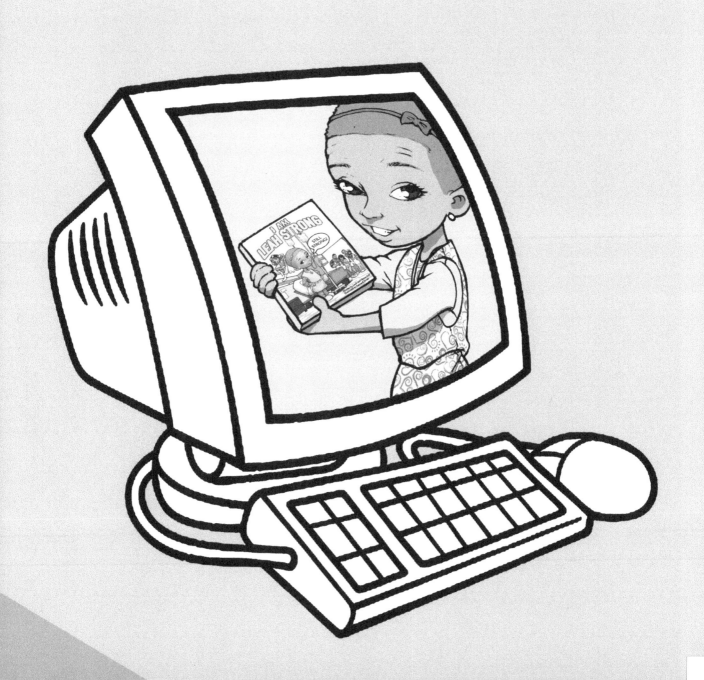

CPSIA information can be obtained at www.ICGtesting.com
Printed in the USA
LVOW02*0408020515

436004LV00002BA/2/P